Obesity Alert

*Cutting Down on Sweets
and Calories, Exercising,
and Minding Your Body*

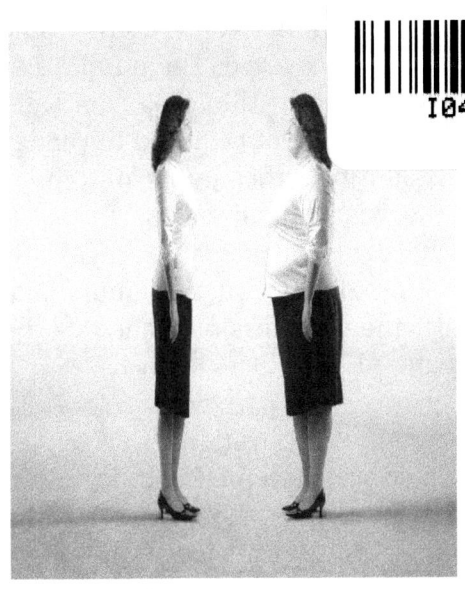

I0420707

By
Fhilcar Faunillan

Fhilcar Faunillan

Obesity Alert

and is universal as so. The presentation of the information is without contract or any type of guarantee assurance.

Table of Contents

INTRODUCTION

I want to thank you and congratulate you for downloading the book, *"Obesity Alert: Cutting Down on Sweets and Calories, Exercising and Minding Your Body"*.

Obesity has become the leading preventable cause of death all over the world. About a third of the adult American population is obese. This just shows how predominant the problem with obesity is. As the number of obese people climbs year after year, this has alarmed various institutions with this dilemma. Have you thought of the possible reasons why obesity is on the rise?

Through the advent of whatever instants – food specifically – the quality of food we take in and our health most especially is compromised. Obesity is prevalent since there is a reduction of manual labor as replaced by machines and new technologies, availability of cheap, unhealthy food sources, and massive patronage of processed as well as fast food.

This book will be your guide in order to combat this problem. Contained in this book are tips on how to curb your sugar addiction, sweat yourself out and shed those extra pounds for complete wellness. Be conscious with your weight as diseases and complications associated with the condition knows no age. Do not wait until a dreadful event in your life would happen and during such time your doctor would recommend that you stop your unhealthy habits. Act now and be one step closer to your health goals.

Thanks again for downloading this book, I hope you enjoy it!

Chapter 1 - Obesity At A Glance

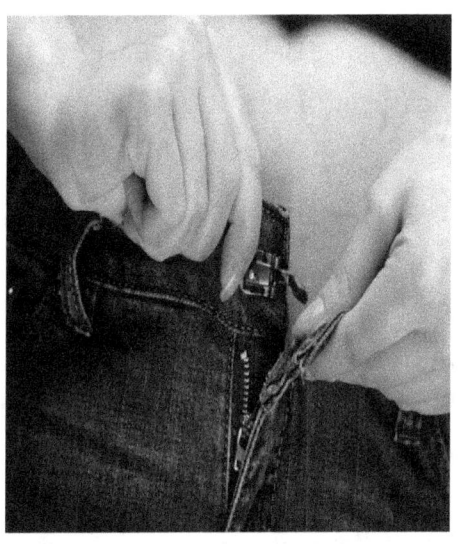

The world has been fighting against obesity since the 1980s but it seems that we are not winning the fight. The number of overweight and obese individuals is even increasing in number.

First off, what is obesity? As a medical condition, obesity results when the body has accumulated excessive fats or in short, has become overweight. This can then cause adverse effects on the body. Obesity is can be tracked by measuring one's Body Mass Index (BMI) or the waist-to-hip ratio.

Over the years, several diets addressing weight problems have risen. It is however proper to stop the drastic dieting and consider a healthy lifestyle that you could follow for the rest of your life. Healthy eating is not just a phase but a lifelong battle for a healthy you. It does not stop on eating alone; having a healthy weight also includes exercise, sleep and other contributory factors.

But before anything, here is how to compute your BMI: BMI is equivalent to your weight (in kilograms) over your height squared (in meters). Your BMI determines whether you are having the right weight for a given height. For those falling under the normal weight category, a BMI of 18.5 to 24.9 is ideal and considered healthy. This is also the BMI range that everyone should maintain. If you are overweight, your BMI is likely to fall within the range of 25 to 29.9. That means that you have gone beyond the standard weight and it is recommended that you lose some weight in order to reach the normal category. Should your waist measurement be high, you are a potential risk of acquiring the so-called lifestyle diseases. The obese category admits of having a BMI that is greater than 30. As your category progresses, the more is the need for you to shed weight. The risk of acquiring diseases associated with obesity is higher than the rest of the categories. For that reason, seeing a doctor is necessary. Thus the need for an active lifestyle as part of having a healthy weight. Regular exercises is a must to slim down. It does not have to be an abrupt heavy exercise. You can start with the simplest household chores and walking.

Depending on the age and gender, the number of calories needed per level of activity varies. Starting with females aged 19 to 30, a sedentary lifestyle needs 2,000 calories. Moderate activities require at least 2,000 to 2,200 while active ones need 2,400. For those that fall under 31 to 50 age bracket, sedentary, moderate and active activities burn 1,800 calories, 2,000 and 2,200 calories, respectively. Older females (51+) only need 1,600, 1800 and 2,000 to 2,200 for sedentary, moderate and active.

As energetic as they are, males need to burn more calories. For the 19 to 30 age bracket, sedentary activities need 2,400 calories, 2,600 to 2,800 for moderate, and 3,000 for active. Those falling under 31 to 50 of age need 2,200 for sedentary, 2,400 to 2,600 for moderate, and 2,800 to 3,000 for active activity level. Older males (50+) have lesser calorie consumption per activity similar to the females. For sedentary, moderate and active activity level, their calorie consumption is 2,000, 2,200 to 2,400 and 2,400 to 2,800, respectively.

For every activity or action that you do, there is a corresponding activity level and calories required. If you eat, go to work and sleep without any activity, you are considered sedentary. Sedentary lifestyle is considered unhealthy. If you do not know your activity level, here is what constitutes your activity level:

- <u>Sedentary:</u> You only do very little physical work or none at all. Those people who do not engage in any type of exercise and spend time sitting, watching TV and sleeping.

- <u>Moderate:</u> You have a moderate activity level when you exercise for about 2 ½ hours per week or you walk around 1.5 to 3 miles per day.

- Active: Congratulations! This is the activity level a healthy person should have. You exercise rigorously at least 2 hours per week or walk more than 3 miles per day.

Now that you are aware how you place in terms of level of activity, you are now able to act upon it. The message here is clear: if you are active, then that is great but if you are sedentary, you have to improve your activity level.

Chapter 2 - The Dangers of Obesity

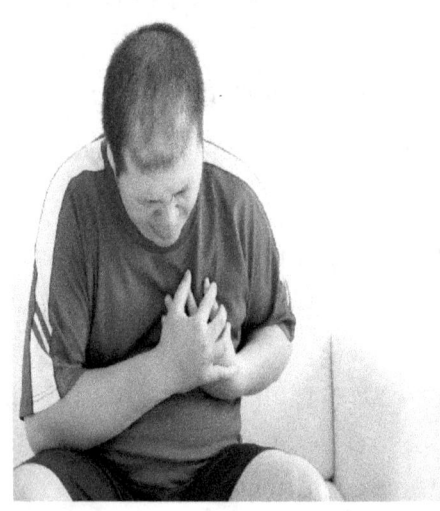

Managing your ideal weight is necessary to lower the risk of various diseases. Obesity is a precursor to many high risk diseases such as atherosclerosis, hypertension, and diabetes among others.

Cardiovascular   disease. Cardiovascular diseases are the leading cause of death around the world. As a bulk of the world's population gets fatter, we are at a higher risk of developing cardiovascular diseases. The movement of our diets from plant-based to animal-based as well as our inactive lifestyle have brought severe consequences to our health.

Why do fats lead us to acquiring cardiovascular diseases? That is because fats especially abdominal fats affect how the body metabolize. Fats affect the blood pressure, blood lipid levels, and interfere with the body's ability to use insulin. Insulin is needed to process the fuel from food. That is why the fatter you get the lesser the body's ability to metabolize.

And the fatter you are, the more likely you are to gain weight.

As to how these fats can pose danger on your health, it can be easily understood. The most common cause of death is due to atherosclerosis. This condition happens the moment fats stick on the arteries causing the latter to harden and become narrow. When the arteries harden and become narrow, blood will have difficulty in passing through. As atherosclerosis progresses, the bump gets bigger thereby creating blockage. The blockage can happen anywhere in your body and may cause problems on the heart, stroke and eventually death.

Diabetes. Diabetes is described as a lifestyle-related metabolic disease that stems up from continued high levels of blood sugar, inadequate insulin production or improper response of the body's cells to insulin. In 2013, over 380 million people are afflicted with diabetes and the numbers are fast growing. The following are the common symptoms that diabetics experience:

- Frequent Urination

- Intense hunger pangs and thirst

- Unusual weight loss

- Numbness and tingling sensation in limbs

- Cuts and bruises that do not heal

- Fatigue

- Sexual dysfunction in males

When you experience most of the symptoms, be sure to test your blood sugar and go to the nearest clinic for a consultation. Make sure that you are able to control your blood sugar levels. You can have high blood sugar levels but not high enough to be considered a diabetic. This is called prediabetes. Those who are pre-diabetics are more likely to develop diabetes in the long run.

Overtime, having too much glucose on your blood can cause complications on your kidneys, eyes and nerves. It may lead to amputation, blindness and even death.

Joint Problems. Overtime, the strain on added weight due to obesity can cause body problems such as joint pains and arthritis. Though this is not a popular effect of obesity, it is as crippling as diabetes and cardiovascular diseases.

Due to the excess weight that the body has to deal with, the joints are rubbed in greater friction causing much more wear and tear of joints, thus the pain. To relieve the joints from extreme pressure, it is advised to keep off the weight at the optimum.

A study by Framingham has proved that when you lose even just about 11 pounds off, you are lowering the risk of developing osteoarthritis by half. If obese and overweight people are suffering from arthritis, shedding off even 5% of their weight can help with the healing, recovery and relief from pain.

It is also suggested to avoid strenuous exercises such as running when suffering from joint pains because the excessive strain and pressure on your joints will worsen the condition. It is recommended to employ exercise routine that are not putting much pressure on your joints such as swimming.

But before starting any exercise regime, please do visit your doctor first. You can ask your doctor the best exercise for you and can recommend someone if you want a trainer. These professionals can help you explain the right mechanics and proper way of exercise.

You should also use exercise materials and tools that are recommended. There are shoes that offer more support to prevent further joint damage. When doing exercise, you should always listen to your body. When you start feeling pain, stop and start again when your body is ready.

It can be deduced that keeping a healthy weight is essential to your joint health.

Chapter 3 - Emotional and Physical Well-Being

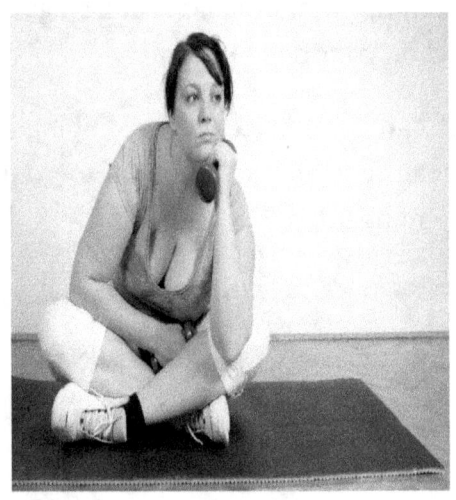

You have probably heard of people who have been happy with their bodies despite having excess weight. Well, good for them for being happy; however, this is not the case for all.

Some may judge heavy-built individuals harshly than those who have slimmer built. Bias, social stigma and discrimination are often suffered by obese and overweight individuals. Those who are still at school may suffer bullying just because they are obese. They are construed as lazy, impulsive, uncontrollable and unattractive.

In the job setting, they are thought of as incompetent and often leave negative impressions on their future employers. This is supported by studies that there is a preconceived notion about medical professionals' impression on obese patients. They think that the obese patients are often associated by doctors with poor hygiene, hostility and dishonesty. Furthermore, other doctors relate them to lack of love or attention, lack of self-control and over-indulgence.

Why do society find obesity as repulsive? Society depicts thinness as the symbol of will power, determination and self-control. These virtues are seen by people as lacking in the obese population. People ascribe obesity as a personal choice and an obese just have to choose to be healthy.

Many suffer from derogatory remarks and teasing due to weight stigma. Fatty, Piggy and other names have been what other people call the obese people. Some may be openly hurt by these names and other brush them off but they have must have been hurt and got irritated. These teasing, name-calling and ridicule are verbal types of bias.

There are some who even suffer from physical types such as grabbing, touching and other abusive overt gestures – many of which have been suffered in school for those obese children. These weight problems may also give them some emotional and psychological setbacks.

As you can deduce form the explanations above, it is not easy to shed off the pounds. Overweight and the obese should not be judged harshly since we do not know their story. They need support and understanding to achieve their weight.

Some of the emotional and psychological setbacks are the very serious and can deeply affect the individual's life and future. Those people who experience weight stigmatization may suffer the following:

- Depression

- Anxiety

- Social Isolation

- Poor Self-Image

- Low self-esteem

Though not every time that an obese person develops these negative effects of weight discrimination, these difficulties are seen higher in those who have higher weight. In this book, we would discuss the emotional and psychological health of those with obesity which is seldom discussed among the consequences of obesity.

Depression. Does depression cause obesity or does obesity cause depression? This is a question that has often plagued scientists. According to obesity studies, it has been shown that obese people are more likely to develop mood disorders such as depression. Since obesity can cause social isolation, poor self-esteem and self-image are contributors to depression.

Depression can cause obesity. Those who are depressed find comfort and solace in food and being alone. Those who are depressed find themselves obese the next year or two. Depressed people also avoid exercise and become sedentary.

Likewise, stigmatization and discrimination are faced by overweight and obese people and these reasons are legitimate. The chronic pain and suffering experienced from diabetes and hypertension are linked with depression. Depression and obesity is a never ending cycle unless acted upon by the individuals and helpful professionals.

Sometimes, obesity seems unending because the emotional and psychological aspect of healing is often neglected. If one aspect of the problem is neglected, there is a chance that the weight loss program you are following may fail. That is why, it is important for those aiming for weight loss to gain support from friends and family. By losing weight, you do not only help yourself physically but also psychologically.

Anxiety. Similar to depression, anxiety plays a role in developing obesity as obesity can cause anxiety. Unlike depression, anxiety disorders' relation with obesity is highly debated by mental health professionals. Though it is quite clear that anxiety alone is not the reason a person develops obesity. It is composed of several factors. Though it is hypothesized that anxiety is a contributor to obesity.

Theoretically, anxiety makes you lose weight since the body is in fight or flight mode. The fight or flight mode makes the body's metabolism faster. But other factors such as cortisol levels, digestion changes and inactivity caused by anxiety contribute to the weight gain.

When cortisol level is constantly at its peaks, cortisol encourages the storage of fat in the stomach causing weight gain. Anxiety can also slow how your body digest food. The longer your stress and anxiety, the more you gain weight.

With stress and anxiety, you are more prone to eat comfort food. Eating is said to be a coping mechanism for those who are anxious. Since the stress is eating away your energy, you will feel fatigue. So when you rest, there is less calories burned that could have keep the weight off.

However, obesity can actually cause you anxiety disorders. Dieting, disease, pain and striving to look good can cause you anxiety. The day-to-day struggle is enough reason to experience stress and anxiety. It is best to tackle your health physically and psychologically.

Social Isolation. A few of us value our 'me-time', but most of the time, we really want to share our time with people close to our hearts. People who live in isolation are more like to lead an unhealthy lifestyle and die earlier than those who don't.

According to 4-year research in Australia, those children who are overweight and obese have been found to have difficulty in establishing peer relationships. Those children often experience a well-documented history of bullying due to weight stigma.

As these children and adolescents experience bullying at school, they may opt to go home-schooled. Those home-schooled have often lesser number of friends and time for socializing, thus, further isolating themselves. These children learn their social skills and develop peer relationships mostly at school, which the home-schooled children miss. When they grow up into adults, they will have difficulty with socializing and gaining and holding peer relationships.

Those who have poor social skills tend to sink further into isolation to avoid awkward situation through social faux pas. They would avoid reunions, parties and keep to herself/himself. Though wanting to experience the niceties of having a great social group, people who isolate themselves are afraid of rejection of peers.

They grow lonely, anxious and alone, they will most likely find comfort with food. Excessive eating will most likely produce excess weight, thus, obesity. When people experience that they are getting heavier, they are more afraid to go out and socialize. It is bad to hear from people how much you got fatter from the last time they saw you. People with gained weight do fear that people would say bad things about themselves when they go out. And comments about weight, no matter how politely said, will hurt. And that is what they try to avoid.

Isolation and obesity is a depressing condition. It would be nice to have people you could share your life with. It does not matter if they are family, friends, colleagues or even just neighbors.

Poor Self-Image. Everyone is unique, beautiful and amazing in their own way. When you are happy with who you are, how you look and what you achieved, then all is well. But this is not the case for everyone. When you are alone, obese and depressed, it is safe to say that you might have poor self-image and low self-esteem.

Body image is how you see yourself. You begin to form your body image through childhood experiences. How you see yourself is also factored by the feedback of family, peers and now, the social media. Overweight and obese people seem to have poor self-image. It may stem from the societal standards that thin is beautiful and how people judge you from the way you look.

Society plays a big role in developing your self-image. When Television Ads and print ads always bombard you with flashy super-skinny models, you will feel insecure towards your body. With the technology today, the online world is a way of lowering your self-image.

The signs that a person has a negative or poor self-image are the following: obsessive mirror checking, self-criticism, constant self-comparison to other people, and envy. These negative thoughts are some of the reasons why people with weight problems are distressed.

The negative self-image also reflect on how people with excess weight stick to fad diets. Fad diets promises fast results with little effort. Who doesn't want to lose weight fast? Adults with weight problems are largely dissatisfied with their bodies. These may stem from constant teasing they receive even as adults.

Most who have poor body-image does not even know they do. They need to have an acceptance of who they are and how they look. And if they wish to lose the excess pounds, they should do so in a healthy way.

Low Self-Esteem. Self-esteem is the overall estimation of ones' worth for happiness. People who have excess weight problem tend to have lower self-esteem in comparison to those with normal weight especially for females. Unlike the other emotional and psychological consequences of obesity, low self-esteem is not a factor in developing obesity. It is a result for being obese.

Self-esteem is developed from childhood and is heavily affected by social support. The huge pressure to fuse and be similar to friends can cause one's self-esteem to plummet. Added to these are the physical standards that are set by the society that are heavily expressed by the media and in the web. Despite the campaign of the media to love yourself in any shape is giving mixed signals when they advertise that being obese or overweight is undesirable.

But susceptibility of having low self-esteem is lower when you have family and friends that are supporting you. When they paint a picture of a good image of yourself, you are more secured of your own worthiness. As long as there are people who gives a person a positive feedback, may it be in career, school, appearance or attitude, it retains a positive self-esteem.

Chapter 4 - The Culprits of Weight Gain

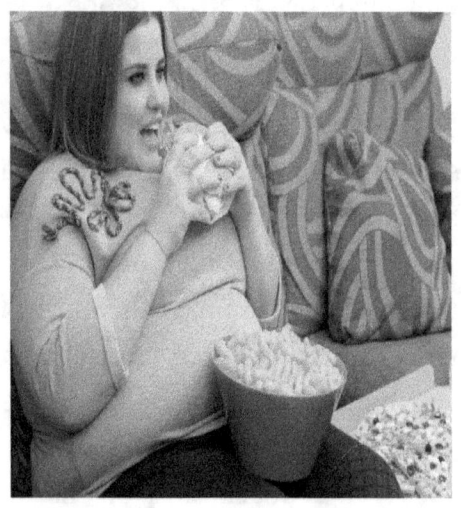

There are varied reasons for weight gain; heredity, environment and lifestyle are major predictors of obesity. These factors contribute to the adding of pounds in the body.

Obesity Alert

Genetics. Some of us are predisposed to a bigger body but not to obesity.

Genetics influence every aspect of lives, physiology, predispositions and even how we adapt. It was originally thought that genetics do not interfere with obesity. But due to the recent advancement in molecular biology, the findings show that there are rare genes that can contribute to obesity risk.

Each person carries a different amount of fat in the body. But some tend to carry more fat than anyone else regardless of the diet observed and exercise undertaken. Moreover, appetite and metabolism is also governed by genetics. Some people are less likely to recognize that they are full. The combination of high fat percentage in the body, healthy appetite, slow metabolism and inability to recognize satiety will result to obesity.

But even if these genetic endowment are present, it is not destiny. This means that despite of having the following genes, it does not mean that you cannot prevent obesity. Many people who have this "obesity gene" did not become obese. Obesity is more of nurture rather than nature.

Diet. Our body needs specified amounts of calories and nutrients to sustain the daily bodily functions. If what we eat is not the right kind and the right amount, it may be the reason for weight gain.

The food that is readily available to the public may not be apt in nourishing the body. For example, fast-food offers unhealthy food at the lowest price but a healthy salad will more like cost thrice than that. The hectic schedule that is brought by the fast paced life makes us prefer for the instants.

What the advertisement offers our eyes are food that are not good for us and our weight such as chips, sweets and sodas. That is why, the generation today have instead chosen what they see is advertisements.

Healthy diet is rarely opted by millions of people because of the availability of instant and unhealthy food. Healthy eating is also hard to follow since it has a reputation of being bland and difficult to make. But if you give having a healthy lifestyle a chance, you will discover that fruits and vegetables are tasty and flavorful.

Sedentary Lifestyle. Having a sedentary lifestyle is considered to be bad for your health. You need to have a very active lifestyle to be considered healthy. When you do not engage in exercise, the muscles that are not used will be atrophied. Moreover, fats that are supposed to be shed off will stay in you.

The modern lifestyle that we lead today does not promote exercise. We stay in front of our televisions or in our computer all day. We are either couch potatoes or internet addicts. The time that is supposed to be spent on physical activity is most of the time spent on things that are unhealthy. Watching television or using the computer is not bad, spending your whole time in front of them is.

Weight gain is not strictly shun because of these factors. There are several other reasons but these are the forefront of having an unhealthy weight. Some may have serious medical complications or a combination of several factors.

Chapter 5 - How to Lose Weight Effectively?

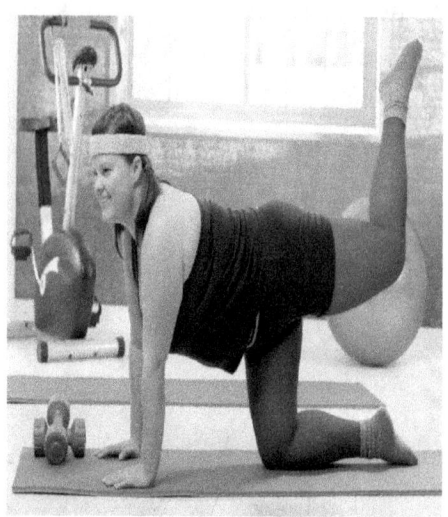

It was emphasized in the previous chapter that psychological and emotional wellness is important in attaining a healthy weight. In this chapter, the aim is to help you to become healthy with your outlook in life.

The first thing you have to consider to change is your diet. Is your diet healthy or do you have to change what you eat? Eating healthy is the first thing you have to ensure to have a healthy weight.

There are different healthy diet concepts that you can adopt. You can use: DASH diet which is recommended by professionals, Vegetarian which consumes only vegetables or low-carb diet. The list of diets continues; you just have to choose the right one for you, as long as it is healthy. To help guide you in having the right food, we would like to discuss the following foods that are essential to your health and how much you should consume every day. And there comes exercise, it is not only for weight loss but also for overall improvement of health.

But before anything else, here are some TIPS in starting your Healthy Eating lifestyle:

1. **Keep a Food and Activity Diary** – before starting a diet, take note of everything that you eat or drink and every activity that you do for a week. It will surprise you how much you eat since there are times that we do not mind what we eat and drink. It will also tell you patterns of your eating habits and how to address this. Like when you watch your late night shows, you cannot keep yourself from grabbing a snack. So next time, you can choose to sleep early instead or have a good reading session.

Having a list will help you track your activity level. In this case, you can keep yourself away from being sedentary. You will also be more aware of tasks and can actually help you organize your schedules.

You can continue the diary even after a lifestyle change; in this way, you can keep yourself away from being tempted to eat more or do less.

2. **Be Informed** – before starting your road to a healthy life, consult your physician first. This is for your own safety. The doctor will check if the drastic changes both on your eating habits and physical activities may not be

suitable for your weight. Being knowledgeable of what you are doing is a great since you will know what to expect.

Research also on the food that are healthy for you. Though it will be discussed here in the later chapter, it may help you further in understanding how healthy living goes. Having facts will make you in control of your situation and know the healthy way of losing weight. It will also explain why there are some diet plans that are not for everyone.

3. **Plan Ahead** –planning your course of action according to what you think is right is the perfect way to do a

change of lifestyle. Planning can help you weigh your options such the food that you will be eating and not eating and the exercise that you will enjoy and have time for.

You can plan what food, activities and beverages that you will cut out from your life. For example, when shopping for food, you will be more aware that there are things that you do not *plan* to eat and will not buy it.

4. **Start with Activities that Can Help You Reach Your Goals** – Just as eating and exercising are indispensable, so are sleep and water. Sleep actually enables you to lose weight.

When you lack sleep, you are more likely to eat more. This is because your body has not achieved the required amount of rest that it needs, therefore, it needs to gain energy from other sources such as food. Lack of sleep can also raise your cortisol levels. Having constant high level of cortisol tends to keep fats in the body especially in the tummy. So start a sleeping plan first so by the time you implement changes, you have a foolproof sleeping pattern.

Water is also an integral part of weight loss. It is recommended that each of us drink at least 8 glasses of water every day. Water regulates our body temperature and flushes fats and toxins out of the body.

Sometimes, we also misidentify thirst and hunger. When hunger is felt, we eat to satisfy ourselves but there are times when we are not actually hungry. Our brain sends signals of thirst but we misidentify it as hunger. So the next time you feel hungry, drink at least a glass of water and wait for 10 minutes. If you are still hungry then that is the right time for you to eat.

So sleep more and drink more for a healthier you. These two activities do not only aid you in losing weight but also in maintaining great health in general.

5. **Have Some Support** – you must gain support from family and friends. You can achieve this by patiently explaining your condition and desire to be healthy. Express clearly how important is this to you. By telling them so, they can help you in your way to weight loss. You can even ask your family to join you in your plans to be healthy and if ever they refuse, ask them to respect your food and activity choices.

Through gaining your family and friends' support, you will be more secured and determined in your endeavors. Since they understood and respect your choice, they will not tempt you to stray from your chosen path.

6. **Do Not Be Discouraged –** there are times that we stray from our path. Do not be discouraged when you commit mistakes. Start again. Always remember that what is important is that you try to right your mistakes. Letting go of your healthy lifestyle just because of a minor incident is a no-no.

Do not think about how hard the changes are but rather think on your health goals. Always remember that in order to achieve something you have to make some sacrifices. You will find ease after some time. The start is always the hardest part of changes but after that, you will find the new you.

Chapter 6 - Emotional, Psychological and Social Preparation for Losing Weight

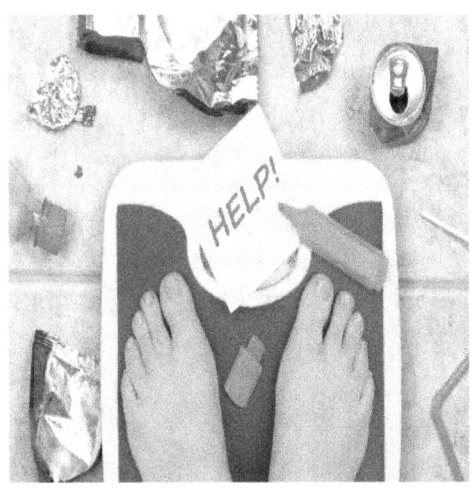

There are times when you think that the physical aspects are the only thing that affects your diet, you are dead wrong. In your journey to healthy eating, especially if you have bad eating habits, you have to be emotionally and psychologically ready for the changes. Remember that when we are emotionally and psychologically stressed, we tend to find comfort in food.

Stress induced comfort eating is counterproductive. Even if you are exercising well, your efforts will become fully ineffective if you have poor eating habits. Most comfort foods are high fat, sugar and even calories. This is very bad for your health and the life ahead of you.

The most important part of having a healthy heart and mind is to be positive – that is, positive of the things to happen, positive in achieving your goals, positive in how you see yourself and finally positive that you will be happy. If you are feeling really helpless, please seek the help of a medical professional. This is because a combination of depressive, low self-esteem and obese factors can cause severe emotional toll. This could lead into suicidal thoughts.

The main reason as to why people want to lose weight is that they want to look good and fit better in clothes. This is why billions of dollars are spent on weight reducing products and services. But rather than focusing on the physical aspect, we should take on a healthier approach. The following tips will discuss how to feel positive and worthy.

- *Do not blame yourself with your weight but accept the fact that you obese are or overweight.* By doing so, you can get rid of the guilt that you have been feeling which in return can add much stress on you.

Accepting the problem is half the battle. Some people experience denial that they are healthy despite being obese or overweight.

- _Identify the source of your problems, stress and anxiety._ Point out what are the causes that brings you to eating too much or exercising too little. These might be circumstances such as stress from work, crisis at home, challenges in relationships or sudden changes in the home or your overall environment. Now that you can identify what is troubling you, you are now aware of your train of thoughts regarding these problems.

- *Analyze your own thoughts.*
  Pay attention to thought patterns that erode your self-esteem. This includes discounting positives and converting into negatives. For example, *"I topped the test because I was lucky"*. Stop these thoughts and accept your achievements and think that you deserve the good things that happened to you. Another pattern is jumping into negative conclusion and dwelling on it. For example, *"I made a mistake and everyone thinks I am loser and up to no good"*. If ever you commit a mistake, acknowledge it, learn from it and let it to. Dwelling on it may lower your spirit and self-esteem. Another

pattern is negative self-talk. For example, *"I cannot do it no matter what"*. What you can do instead is to encourage yourself that you can do better. You will never know whether you can do it or not if you do not give it a try.

- *Believe in yourself.* If you hear negative things pertaining your weight, accept them but do not keep them to heart. You know that you are overweight or obese, that is why you are choosing a healthy lifestyle because you want to shed off those pounds. You should believe that your health endeavors will be successful. If you refuse to think that you will succeed, you will more likely fail.

- *Have a creative visualization.* This is a technique that use mental images that can help you achieve your goals. If your goal is losing weight, you can visualize yourself as someone who is slimmer, healthier and fitter. Imagine a long life ahead of you without the debilitating consequential disease due to obesity. Visualize yourself fitting into clothes. Think of how weight related teasing will stop. Just focus on the positive outcomes of your lifestyle change to inspire you to succeed.

- *Have some positive list.* This is a great way to emphasize your own capacity, traits and features in a positive way. Make one for your strength, one for your achievements and one for the things that you admire about yourself. You can ask family and friends in completing your list. You might be surprised about the traits that they like in you. You should always read them and place them in your room that easily be seen.

- *Have some social support.* No man or woman is here on earth to be alone. Humans are social creatures. That is why we need family and friends in order to succeed. Tell your family and friends about your plans. Ask them their opinions and suggestions. They might as well have similar goals with you and join you on the road to healthy living. Bond with the people you hold very dear and at the same time, try to meet new people. It will widen your social circle as well as your horizons. Remember, avoid places and people that will make you feel bad about yourself and tempt you to do things against your will.

When you are depressed or think that you are depressed, it is best that you seek out the help of your doctor. Depression is a serious case that can cause severe scars psychologically and emotionally.

Chapter 7 - What to Eat?

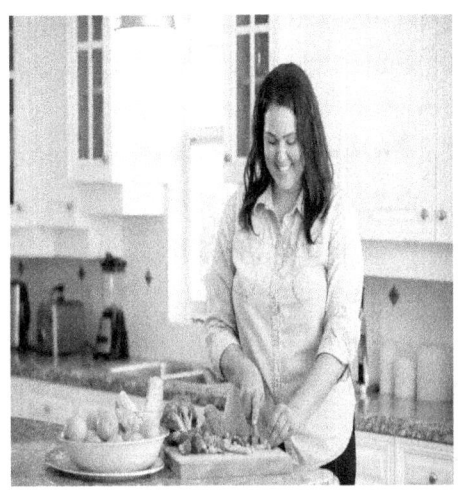

There are several diets available that promises you to lose weight fast and for good. As already mentioned, we should aim to make our eating practices not a temporary fix but a permanent one throughout our lifetime. If you think that eating to shed off the pounds is temporary, you might gain the pounds again when you attain your desired weight.

You must know that the food you take is for our body's daily needs such as breathing, pumping blood around the body, thinking and other bodily involuntary functions. The body burns the food for other voluntary actions such as walking, talking, jumping, and others. The key to weight loss is to burn the calories more than the calories from the food that you eat.

It is not recommended to follow those fad diets. The faster weight loss it promises, the more you have to be wary of it. For example, micro-diet have been popular for those who wanted to shed off pounds fast. Micro-diets are diets where you consume only 350 calories a day. This is bad for the body since the body needs at least 1500 calories for women and 2000 calories for men.

Obesity Alert

Starving is really bad for those who are trying to lose weight. Apart from the fact that you are denying your body of the right nourishments, starving lowers the body metabolism. When you starve, the body actually thinks that you are really starving and takes appropriate action. This is why even those who eat less than 1000 calories still gain weight.

While the amount of calories present in food is important, the quality of its food source is equally important. The food must have the nutrients that you need. You must eat a variety of food to obtain the right nourishment. You need carbohydrates, protein, fruits, vegetables and very little sugar and fats. This book emphasizes on "HEALTHY LIFESTYLE".

Before anything, you should know the importance of the following nutrients and the amount you should consume them. These are major sources of nutrients for the body.

Carbohydrates

Carbohydrates have the reputation of destroying you weight. Fad diets are now fearing the evil carbohydrates. Carbohydrates are now considered to be bad for your waist. But that is not entirely true. Carbohydrates are essential to our diet since it provides the necessary energy for our daily function. But too much of carbs is dangerous to your weight. That is why you just have to choose the right type of carbohydrates and the amount that you have to consume daily.

Obesity Alert

There are three types of carbohydrates: complex carbohydrate or starch, sugar and fiber. When you estimate the amount of carbohydrate you consume daily, you just have included all types of carbohydrates.

It is easy to separate the good from the bad. You can reap benefits by consuming carbohydrates that is full of fiber. These carbohydrates are slowly absorbed by the body, avoiding sudden spikes in the blood sugar levels. Remember, constant high blood sugar levels can lead to diabetes.

The foods that are high in fiber include whole grains, fruits and vegetables. These foods are also high in complex carbohydrates that give you energy to function daily. To avoid consuming unhealthy food, you should avoid processed carbohydrates such as doughnuts, fries, candies and soda. These foods have high sugar content which is not good for a healthy diet.

For a healthy adult, 25-30 grams of fiber is needed. Sugar should be consumed at the very least. You can have high sugar foods sparingly.

Protein from Meat and Plant Sources

Protein is an important part of any healthy diet plan. Proteins are the building blocks of the body and is essential in any bodily function. Proteins take longer to digest and metabolize so you feel full longer.

You can have protein from animal and plant sources. But you need to consider the type of proteins you are to consume. Animal meat has fats in it, you have to find parts that have very low fats. Consumption therefore of lean meat is always recommended as animal fats are not really healthy for you.

The amount of protein you need to consume depends on your age, sex and level of physical activity. But an average adult can consume around 5-6 ounces of lean meat or other sources, given that you have a moderate activity level. If you exercise extensively, you are allowed to consume more.

Fruits and Vegetables

It is of common knowledge that vegetables are healthy for you. The problem is that a lot people actually do not like vegetables. I know a lot who only consume potato fries and no other. Vegetables are judged as unpalatable. But this is not true; several dishes made with vegetables are mouth-watering and sumptuous.

Vegetables are the best sources of nutrients such as fiber, potassium, foliate, and Vitamins A, C, and E. Many of these vegetables are known to provide additional benefits that can cause prevention of several serious diseases that they are considered super-foods. These super-foods are collier, spinach, tomatoes and garlic. You have to make sure that you include them in your plate.

Fruits on the other hand are willingly consumed by many. They are good sources of vitamins and minerals such as A and C. Continuous consumption of fruits can protect you from the risk of having chronic diseases.

Health professionals recommend that you to consume fruits and vegetables daily. Half of your plate should be fruits and vegetables. You are encouraged to eat 3-4 cups of them daily. You can prepare them in variety of ways depending on the taste that you want.

I will provide you with examples per food group and the recommended amount to consume to serve as your guide. It can be seen that healthy living actually offers a lot of varieties with food. The servings follow the 2000 average calorie daily requirement. This daily requirement of a person vary with gender and age. In the first chapter, you learned the amount of calories you have to consume. Through this guide, food portions can now be easily estimated and prepared.

1. **Grains**

   For grains (whole wheat bread, whole wheat pita bread, brown rice, whole wheat pasta, wholegrain bagel and cereal) which are the main sources of fiber, the recommended daily serving is 6-8. As serving guide, you can have a cup of cereal, or half cup of cooked pasta, or a slice of bread.

2. **Vegetables and fruits**

   These are the best sources of potassium, magnesium, fiber, and other vitamins and minerals. For vegetables, you can have broccoli, carrots, spinach, squash, tomatoes, and peas.

Fruit sources can include apple, banana, dates, grapefruit, mangoes, pineapples, and strawberries. The recommended daily serving is 4-5 for both vegetables and fruits. For instance, you can have half cup of vegetables or a cup of green leafy vegetables. Also, half cup of fresh fruit or a medium fruit is best included in every meal.

3. Fat-free Milk and Dairy

A great source of calcium and protein, emphasis is always stressed on fat-free or low fat milk and dairy products. Have 2-3 servings per day. You can consume either a cup of fat-free or low-fat milk or yogurt or an ounce and a half of low-fat cheese.

4. Lean Meat

Lean meat is a great source of protein. For poultry sources, you can remove the skin. The recommended daily serving is 6 or less. You can consume an ounce of cooked meat, poultry, beef, fish, or an egg.

5. Nuts, Seeds, and Legumes

While these (almonds, mixed nuts, hazelnuts, kidney beans, split peas, walnuts, peanuts and sunflower seeds) are very rich sources of energy, protein, magnesium and fiber, these should be consumed in moderation. You need to have 4-5 servings per week only. You can consume one-third cup of nuts, or half a cup of cooked legumes, or 2 tablespoons of peanut butter.

6. Essential Fats and Oils

Among the best sources of fats and oils are soft margarine, canola oil, olive oil, low-fat mayonnaise, and light salad dressing. You can consume 2-3 servings per day. Have any of these: a teaspoon of margarine, a teaspoon of vegetable oil, one tablespoon of mayonnaise, or 2 tablespoons of salad dressing.

7. Sweets and Added Sugar

Sugar, hard candy, fruit punch, sorbet, and maple syrup can be low in fat and a good source of added energy. However, these should also be taken in moderation of about less than 5 servings per week. You can consume a tablespoon of sugar, a cup of lemonade, or half cup of gelatin or sorbet.

Most of us know which healthy foods to eat including the suggested amounts to consume but more often than not, we ignore such and still opt to eat those unhealthy, salty and sugary foods. Why is that so? One reason could be that unhealthy foods are tastier while healthy foods are bland. This is not really true. What you taste in instant food is just the salt but home-cooked healthy dishes actually offer a more palatable choice.

The right combination of food is encourage in order to have a more nutritious meal. If you eat burger and fries for dinner, it does not provide you the right amount of nutrients. It mostly contain fats, bad carbohydrates and protein. This is not the way for a healthy lifestyle.

You can always experiment in your meals. You can choose any combination of fruits, vegetables protein carbs, and others. Below are some recipes to guide you in cooking healthily. These recipes are also found in fast food restaurants but these are prepared with your health in mind.

Recipe #1   Yoghurt with Honey and Nuts

Serving: 1
Ingredients:
2 tablespoons walnut (halves)
1 cup of Greek yoghurt
1 teaspoon of honey

Procedure:
1. Toast walnut in a skillet until fragrant. Cool then chop.
2. In a bowl, scoop the yoghurt. Top the honey and sprinkle the walnut.

Recipe #2   Miso Soup with Tofu

Serving: 1
Ingredients:
2 strands dried wakame (edible seaweed)
1 cup low-sodium chicken broth
½ cup chopped baby spinach
½ cup tofu
½ tablespoon miso

Procedure:

1. In a large bowl, place the wakame and add hot water. Cover until the wakame is soft. Remove the tough center rib and coarsely chop.

2. Boil the broth in a saucepan and then add the wakame. In a low heat, cover and simmer until tender. Add the spinach and tofu until the spinach begins to wilt. Remove from heat.

3. Combine ¾ of the hot broth with the miso soup in a small bowl until blended. Stir into the soup and serve.

Recipe #3   Linguine Carbonara

Servings: 2-3
Ingredients:
½ pound linguine
1 ounce thinly sliced chopped pancetta
2 teaspoons olive oil
1 chopped onion
1 egg
¼ cup nonfat sour cream
¼ cup grated Parmesan cheese
½ teaspoon ground black pepper

Procedure:

1. Cook the linguine according to package directions. Reserve 2 tablespoons of the cooking liquid. Return the linguine and reserved liquid to the cooking pot; cover and keep warm.

2. Cook the pancetta in a non-stick skillet in medium-high heat until crisp. Transfer the pancetta to a plate and set aside.

3. Heat the oil in the same skillet and then add the onion. Cook and occasionally turn until it is until golden.

4. Mix the egg, sour cream, Parmesan and pepper in a small bowl. Add the cooked onion and the egg mixture in the linguine. Cook over low heat just until heated. Serve with sprinkled pancetta.

Recipe #4   Coconut Rice Pudding

Servings: 6
Ingredients:

3 cups light coconut milk
¾ cup fat-free milk
½ cup long-grain rice
¼ cup brown sugar
1 teaspoon vanilla extract
½ teaspoon ground cinnamon

Procedure:

1. In a medium saucepan, combine coconut milk, milk, rice and sugar. Bring to simmer, cover and cook over low heat until the rice is tender and the mixture is creamy.
2. Remove from the heat and stir in the vanilla extract.
3. Serve the pudding warm or chilled.

Recipe #5   Kung Pao Shrimp

Servings: 4
Ingredients:
¼ c. rice wine or sake
1 tsp. Asian (dark) sesame oil
¾ c. chicken broth (low sodium)
1 tbsp. chill-garlic sauce
2 tbsp. soy sauce
1 ½ tbsp. honey
1 tbsp. cornstarch

2 tsp. canola oil
1 lb. medium-sized shrimp, peeled and deveined
4 c. broccoli florets
3 scallions, chopped
2 tbsp. freshly peeled ginger, minced
2 cloves garlic, minced
1 can of bamboo shoots, drained

Procedure:
1. In a bowl, combine the honey, broth, soy sauce, chili-garlic sauce, sesame, oil rice wine or sake, and cornstarch.
2. Heat a non-stick wok or a large, deep skillet over medium-high heat. Swirl in the canola oil, and then add the shrimp. Stir-fry until opaque in the center and transfer to the plate.
3. Add the scallions, ginger, and garlic; stir-fry until fragrant. Add the broccoli florets and bamboo shoots and stir-fry until crisp-tender. Add the broth mixture and the shrimp.

4. Cook while constantly stirring until the mixture boils down and thickens.
5. Serve and enjoy.

Recipe #6   Whole-Wheat Cranberry Scones

Servings: 10
Ingredients:
1 1/3 cups all-purpose flour
2/3 cup whole-wheat flour
¼ cup brown sugar
2 ½ teaspoon baking soda
½ teaspoon salt
3 tablespoons butter cut in small pieces
¼ cup sweetened cranberries
2 teaspoons grated orange rind
1 large lightly beaten egg
½ cup fat-free buttermilk
1 teaspoon confectioner's sugar

Procedure:
1. Preheat the oven to 375 Fahrenheit. Line the baking sheet with wax paper.

2. In a large bowl, mix in the all-purpose flour, whole-wheat flour, granulated sugar, baking powder, baking soda and salt. Cut in the batter with a pastry blender until the mixture is crumbly.

3. Using a fork, stir in the cranberries and the orange rind. Add the egg and the buttermilk and stir with fork until the dry ingredients are moist. Gather the mixture into a ball, put in the baking sheet and pat into a 7-inch circle. Using a knife dipped in flour, cut the dough into 10 wedges. Do not separate he wedges.

4. Bake until it becomes golden and the toothpick inserted in the center comes out clean. Transfer into a rack.

5. Add the confectioner's sugar on the top and cut with a serrated knife.

6. Serve warm.

Recipe #7   Squash Pie
Servings: 4

Ingredients:
1 tablespoon extra-virgin olive oil
1 chopped onion
1 ½ pounds zucchini, trimmed, grated and squeezed dry
1 ½ cups cooked rice
¾ cup crumbled reduced-fat feta cheese
1/3 cup chopped fresh mint
1/3 cup chopped fresh parsley
1 large lightly beaten egg
¼ teaspoon salt
1/8 teaspoon freshly ground pepper
6 sheets phyllo dough, thawed according to package directions

Procedure:
1. Preheat oven to 350 degrees Fahrenheit. Spray a 7 x 11-inch baking dish with a non-stick low-fat spray; set aside.
2. Heat a large non-stick skillet over medium-high heat for the filling. Swirl in a teaspoon of oil and then add the onion. Cook until softened and transfer to a bowl. Swirl the remaining oil into the skillet, then add the zucchini. Cook

until the liquid from the zucchini evaporates.

3. Add the cooked zucchini to the bowl with onions. Mix in the rice, parsley, feta, mint, egg, salt and pepper.

4. Place one sheet of phyllo with the long side facing you. Lightly spray the phyllo sheet with non-stick spray; top with the second phyllo sheet and then spray with the non-stick spray. Repeat with the remaining phyllo sheets. With a sharp knife, cut the sheet in half, crosswise. Put the half of the phyllo sheets at the bottom of the baking pan. Spread the mixed filling on the top and then cover with the remaining half of the phyllo sheets.

5. Bake until the phyllo is golden and the filling is hot.

Chapter 8 - Move It and Be Active

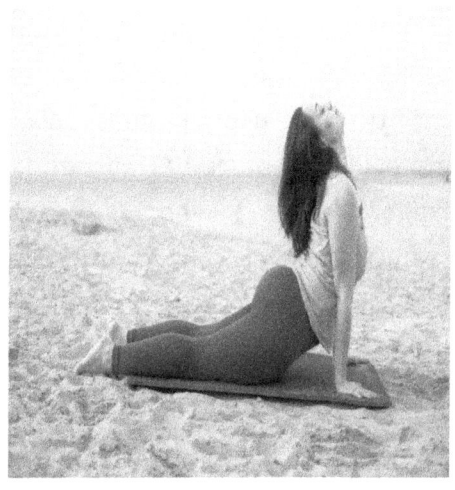

Exercise can be best described as a physical activity that enhances or maintains the physical, emotional, psychological and overall wellness. Exercise strengthens the muscles and cardiovascular system and promotes weight loss and overall health. Exercise can actually help your body defend you from heart and cardiovascular diseases, obesity, diabetes, and depression among others.

There are different types of exercises. *Aerobic exercise* is an activity that uses large muscles and causes your body to use more oxygen than when resting. Examples of aerobic exercises are cycling, running, swimming and hiking. *Anaerobic exercise* or strength training is an activity that is used for firming, strengthening and toning the muscles. It can also improve the balance, coordination and bone strength. Examples of anaerobic exercise would be push-ups, lunges and biceps curls. Lastly, *flexibility* is when your muscles are stretched and lengthen. An example is the sport gymnastics that is heavily reliant of the athlete's flexibility.

An obese person needs special care when it comes to exercise. Since overweight and obese persons carry more weight, they need to go through exercises that are not detrimental to their health.

Here are tips that can help you when exercising:

- _Seek the advice of a doctor before beginning any exercise regimen._ With that, you will be able to choose the right kind of exercise as well as learn the dangers of performing strenuous exercises. Your doctor may tell you to avoid exercises that may potentially strain your joints heavily such as running and jumping. Doctors would highly recommend swimming, which is likewise a great exercise but can put a little pressure on your joints. With that, you are ensured that your joints will be safe from any injury.

- _Consider professional help by hiring a personal trainer._ Trainers are great when you plan to exercise. They will be able to tell you the right way to perform exercise as well as the right amount of exercise you are able to perform. Furthermore, having a trainer improves the quality of your exercise since he/she will encourage you not to stop and push yourself to the limit.

- _Make sure that you eat the right kind and amount of food._ If you exercise and get starved, you might feel light-headed and even worse, experience what you call a *black-out.* Food is necessary for energy. Also, ensure that you are hydrated. Drink plenty of water to replace the water you will lose when you exercise.

- *Find a comfortable place to exercise.* If you do not feel comfortable exercising in a gym then you can opt to do it outdoors.

- *Avoid machines.* Machines are made without the consideration for those who are obese. Obese people are having difficulty in operating machines. It is best to use an exercise plan that may be easier for you to follow. As you progress in your exercise plan, the intensity and duration can increase.

- _Do not forget to warm up._ Warming up before starting your exercise warms your muscle tissues, tendons and ligaments. Warming up is priming your muscles for the work they are about to do. By doing so, potential injuries can be avoided. It has been reported that those who warm up before performing an exercise are less prone to injuries.

- _Wear the proper attire and use proper equipment._ The right clothes and shoes offer you a great deal of support and comfort. Usage of equipment in the right way also ensures your safety from injuries.

- *Join sports.* Playing a sport that you enjoy is a great avenue for a new passion and new friends. You might meet friends you will treasure, experience the spirit of competition, and still have the benefits of an exercise.

Below are some fundamental exercises that you might want to start with. They are easy to follow yet a great exercise.

Squats

1. When trying to squat, most of us have the knees protrude far over the toes, the butt goes straight down, and the heels come off the floor.

97

To perform the perfect squat, you should hinge your hips so that your butt moves backwards during the downward phase of the squat. Your knees will no longer protrude well over your toes. Finally, the pressure of the squat will be on your heels instead on your toes and you will be able to get more depth to your squat.

2. People tend to make mistakes when they squat that is by either rounding their necks, or looking down to the ground. By doing these, the spinal alignment is thrown off which makes

the squat a very dangerous exercise especially if you are overweight or obese.

3. The most important thing to consider when squatting is making sure your spine is in proper alignment. Keep your shoulder backwards and your chest out and your lower back will most likely have the correct natural curve. When you round your shoulders and sink your chest in, your spinal alignment will be thrown off.

4. The bottom of the spine has a slight arch. You should keep your lower back flat to slightly arch as you squat.

Hyper-extending your lower back through arching too much, or rounding your back can give significant pressure on your inter-vertebral discs, which are gel like cushions that protect each vertebrae. If the disc bursts because of too much pressure, a portion of the spinal disc pushes outside its normal boundary. This so-called herniated disc may require surgery to repair. It can't be emphasized enough to make sure your lower back is flat to slightly arched throughout the entire squat movement.

5. When squatting, use an athletic stance to be sure your knees are bent slightly, with your feet firmly planted on the ground and toes pointed slightly outwards. This way, your posture is stabilized. The wider you put your feet, the more it works your glutes and hamstring, and the easier it will be to stabilize. The closer you put your feet, the more your quadriceps will be emphasized.

6. Breathing is very important for achieving the perfect squat in particular because it is a challenging exercise.

Improper breathing can make you light headed, or nauseous, and in extreme cases, faint.

As you bring yourself lower to the ground, remember to take a deep breath in, then as you are pushing up, breath out forcefully. Always keep this breathing pattern. Towards the last few repetitions, you may consider taking a few extra breaths at the top of the squat position as you are standing for some extra energy.

7. The depths of your squats depend on the flexibility of your hips as well as the strength of

your legs. Remember that the lower you go the better since it stretches more muscles in your body. Be careful in performing this exercise especially if you are carrying weight.

Step It Up

Beginner:

1. Find a step or bench that when you place your foot on it, your knee is at a 90-degree angle. Make sure that the bench that you choose is sturdy enough to hold your weight.

2. To start, step up leading with the right foot and then the left, bringing both feet onto the bench.

3. Return to the first position by having the right foot to step down to the floor, then the left, until ending with both feet on the ground.

4. Complete 20 steps and start another 20 steps using your left foot as lead.

Intermediate:

Find a step or bench so that when you place your foot on it, your knee is at a 90-degree angle. Make sure that the bench that you choose is sturdy enough to hold your weight.

1. Put your left foot on the bench.

2. Bring your right foot up and lift the right leg to a 90-degree angle, lower your right foot down to tap the floor. Make sure your left foot never moves

as you bend and straighten your right knee. This completes one rep.

3. Complete 20 reps on each leg.

Push-ups with Elevated Feet

1. Lie on the floor, face down and place your hands about 36 inches apart from each other holding your torso up at arms' length.

2. Place your toes on top of a flat bench. This will allow your body to be elevated. Note: The higher the elevation of the flat bench, the higher the resistance of the exercise is.

3. Lower yourself slowly until your chest is almost touching the floor as you inhale.

4. Using your pectoral muscles, press your upper body back up to the starting position and squeeze your chest. Breathe out as you perform this step.

5. After a second, pause at the contracted position, repeat the movement for the prescribed amount of repetitions.

CONCLUSION

Thank you again for downloading this book!

You have discovered the different aspects of obesity – form its causes to its cure. Now that you are equipped with knowledge in understanding and dealing with obesity, you are more capable of gaining the weight that you desired. Always remember that obesity is not only based on the physical factors but also the emotional and psychological ones.

It would be great to witness your metamorphosis: *from an obese or overweight individual, beautifully transformed into a healthy, fit and happy person that you long to be for years.* I simply hope that you maintain whatever that you gain from reading this book. Now, what it takes is just to apply what you learned, start the change and see the new you.

The road to healthy living is never easy. But you have learned what is needed to be done in order to be healthy. You can now be a healthy person through your will and determination. Let no mistakes and hurdles stop you from achieving the goals that you have set for yourself. Remember to trust in yourself. You are amazing, unique and worthy.

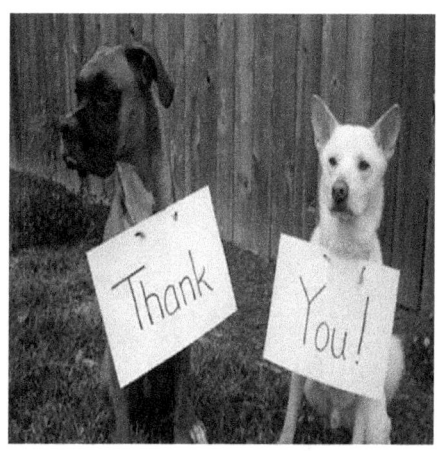

Finally, if you enjoyed this book, then I'd like to ask you for a favor, would you be kind enough to leave a review for this book on Amazon? It'd be greatly appreciated!

Thank you and good luck!